Rise Above Jet Lag

*Thrive in Any Time Zone
with Expert Strategies*

Blake Brook

Copyright © Blake Brook, 2023.

Table of Contents

Introduction

The Jet Lag Phenomenon and its Impact on Well-being

Jet lag, an all-too-familiar experience for frequent travelers, can take a toll on our bodies and minds, leaving us feeling fatigued, disoriented, and struggling to adjust to new time zones. Whether you're a business traveler, an adventure seeker, or simply embarking on a much-needed vacation, the effects of jet lag can hinder your ability to fully enjoy your travel experience and perform at your best.

In this book, "Rise Above Jet Lag: Thrive in Any Time Zone with Expert Strategies," we delve into the science, challenges, and effective solutions for conquering jet lag. With insights from experienced travelers and sleep experts, we provide a comprehensive guide to help you rise above the struggles of jet lag and embrace a journey of vitality and well-being, regardless of the time zone.

Throughout the pages of this book, you will gain a deep understanding of the factors contributing to jet lag and its impact on your body's circadian rhythms. We will explore the art of pre-travel preparation, equipping you with invaluable strategies to optimize your sleep patterns, physical state, and mental well-being prior to departure.

Once on board, you'll discover a range of in-flight strategies to promote rest and recovery, enabling you to arrive at your destination feeling refreshed and ready to conquer the challenges ahead. We will unravel the secrets of time zone transition, offering expert techniques to synchronize your body's internal clock with the new environment, minimizing the disruption to your sleep and energy levels.

But it doesn't stop there. This book goes beyond the basics of sleep and jet lag recovery, delving into the realms of nutrition, hydration, and active strategies that support your body's ability to adapt and thrive in any time zone. You'll uncover the power of natural remedies and supplements, harnessing their potential to alleviate jet lag symptoms and boost your overall well-being.

Moreover, we recognize the demands of modern life and the importance of maintaining productivity and performance while combating jet lag. We provide practical tips and techniques to help you stay focused, accomplish your goals, and make the most of your travel experience, whether it's for business or pleasure.

Rise Above Jet Lag

"Rise Above Jet Lag" is not just a temporary fix; it's a comprehensive guide for long-term jet lag prevention and management. We explore sustainable lifestyle habits and routines that will empower you to seamlessly integrate travel and time zone adjustments into your daily life, ensuring optimal well-being and vitality no matter where your adventures take you.

Get ready to unlock the secrets to conquering jet lag and embrace a life of boundless energy and adventure. Let's rise above jet lag together and thrive in any time zone!

Chapter 1

Understanding Jet Lag

Exploring the Science Behind Jet Lag and Its Effects on the Body and Mind

Jet lag is a phenomenon that has plagued travelers for decades. It occurs when our internal body clock, also known as the circadian rhythm, becomes desynchronized with the external environment due to rapid travel across multiple time zones. The resulting misalignment between our internal clock and the local time can have significant effects on our body and mind, leading to fatigue, sleep disturbances, mood swings, and decreased cognitive function. In this chapter, we will delve deep into the science behind jet lag, unraveling its mechanisms and understanding how it affects our overall well-being.

The Circadian Rhythm:

To understand jet lag, we must first grasp the concept of the circadian rhythm. Our bodies operate on a natural 24-hour cycle, influenced by various internal and external factors. This internal clock regulates our sleep-wake cycle, hormone production, body temperature, and other physiological processes. The circadian rhythm is primarily regulated by a small region in the brain called the suprachiasmatic nucleus (SCN), which responds to environmental cues such as light and darkness.

Disruption of the Circadian Rhythm:

When we travel across time zones, our circadian rhythm struggles to adjust to the new schedule imposed by the local time. This misalignment occurs because our bodies are accustomed to a particular routine based on our home time zone. The sudden shift can lead to confusion and disarray within our biological processes, resulting in the symptoms commonly associated with jet lag.

Effects of Jet Lag on the Body:

Jet lag can manifest in various ways and affect different bodily functions. One of the primary effects is sleep disturbances. Our bodies struggle to adapt to the new sleep schedule, leading to difficulty falling asleep, frequent awakenings during the night, and a general feeling of unrest. This disruption of sleep patterns can result in daytime fatigue, decreased alertness, and impaired cognitive performance.

Additionally, jet lag can impact our digestive system, leading to appetite changes, gastrointestinal discomfort, and irregular bowel movements. Hormonal imbalances may also occur, affecting the regulation of hunger, satiety, and other metabolic processes. The immune system can be weakened, making travelers more susceptible to illnesses and infections.

Effects of Jet Lag on the Mind:

Beyond the physical symptoms, jet lag can also have a profound impact on our mental well-being. Many individuals experience mood swings, irritability, and difficulty concentrating. The cognitive effects of jet lag can hinder our ability to perform tasks that require focus, memory, and problem-solving skills. These mental challenges can be particularly problematic for business travelers or those who need to be at their best immediately upon arrival.

Jet Lag and Shift Work:

While jet lag is commonly associated with travel, it shares similarities with another phenomenon known as shift work sleep disorder. Individuals who work night shifts or frequently rotate between different shifts often experience similar disruptions in their circadian rhythm, leading to similar symptoms as those caused by jet lag. Understanding the similarities and differences between these two conditions can provide valuable insights into the management and mitigation of jet lag.

Mitigating the Effects of Jet Lag:

While jet lag cannot be completely eliminated, there are strategies and techniques that can help mitigate its effects and facilitate a smoother transition. In the following chapters, we will explore pre-travel preparations, in-flight strategies, sleep optimization techniques, nutrition and hydration considerations, and more. By implementing these approaches, travelers can significantly reduce the severity and duration of jet lag symptoms, allowing for a more enjoyable and productive travel experience.

Factors That Contribute to the Severity of Jet Lag Symptoms

Jet lag affects individuals to varying degrees, with some people experiencing milder symptoms while others struggle with more severe disruptions to their well-being. The severity of jet lag symptoms can be influenced by several factors, including individual differences, travel-related factors, and lifestyle choices. In this chapter, we will explore these factors in depth to gain a better understanding of why some individuals may be more susceptible to the effects of jet lag than others.

Individual Differences:

One of the key factors that contribute to the severity of jet lag symptoms is individual differences in circadian rhythm regulation. Some people naturally have a more flexible internal clock, allowing them to adapt more easily to new time zones and minimize the impact of jet lag. On the other hand, individuals with a more rigid circadian rhythm may struggle more when faced with rapid time zone changes. Genetic factors and age can also play a role in how individuals respond to jet lag.

Travel-Related Factors:

The specifics of travel, such as the number of time zones crossed, the direction of travel, and the duration of the journey, can influence the severity of jet lag symptoms. The more time zones crossed, the greater the disruption to the body's internal clock. Eastward travel tends to be more challenging for most individuals, as it requires adjusting to an earlier time zone, which can be more difficult than adapting to a later time zone when traveling westward. Longer flights and multiple layovers can also add to the overall fatigue and exacerbate jet lag symptoms.

Sleep Deprivation:

Lack of adequate sleep prior to travel can intensify the impact of jet lag. Starting a trip already sleep-deprived can make it harder for the body to adjust to the new time zone and recover from the effects of jet lag. It is crucial to prioritize quality sleep in the days leading up to travel to minimize the severity of symptoms.

Stress and Anxiety:

The stress and anxiety associated with travel can amplify the effects of jet lag. High levels of stress can disrupt sleep patterns and make it more challenging for the body to adapt to a new time zone. Taking steps to manage stress, such as practicing relaxation techniques, engaging in mindfulness exercises, or seeking support, can help mitigate the impact of jet lag.

Lifestyle Choices:

Certain lifestyle choices can either alleviate or exacerbate the severity of jet lag symptoms. Factors such as alcohol consumption, caffeine intake, and physical activity levels can influence the body's ability to adjust to a new time zone. Excessive alcohol consumption and high caffeine intake can disrupt sleep patterns and worsen jet lag symptoms. Engaging in regular physical activity can help regulate the body's circadian rhythm and promote better sleep quality, thus aiding in the adjustment to a new time zone.

Preparation and Planning:

The level of preparation and planning before and during travel can also impact the severity of jet lag symptoms. Taking proactive steps, such as gradually adjusting sleep schedules in the days leading up to travel, aligning meal times with the destination's time zone, and exposing oneself to natural light at appropriate times, can help the body adapt more smoothly to the new environment.

Chapter 2

Pre-Travel Preparation

Strategies for Adjusting Your Sleep Schedule and Routines Before Departure

One of the key factors in minimizing the impact of jet lag is preparing your body and mind for the upcoming time zone change. By making deliberate adjustments to your sleep schedule and routines before departure, you can help synchronize your internal body clock with the destination's time zone, making it easier to adapt and reduce the severity of jet lag symptoms. In this chapter, we will explore various strategies and techniques for pre-travel preparation that can help optimize your sleep and promote a smoother transition to a new time zone.

Understanding Your Destination:

The first step in pre-travel preparation is gaining a thorough understanding of your destination's time zone. Familiarize yourself with the time difference and the local customs regarding sleep and meal times. This information will serve as a foundation for planning and adjusting your sleep schedule accordingly.

Gradual Adjustment:

Rather than abruptly changing your sleep schedule on the day of departure, it is beneficial to make gradual adjustments in the days leading up to your trip. Start by shifting your bedtime and wake-up time by 15 to 30 minutes each day, moving closer to the schedule of your destination. This gradual adjustment helps ease your body into the new time zone and minimizes the shock of sudden changes.

Light Exposure:

Light exposure plays a crucial role in regulating the body's circadian rhythm. Use natural light to your advantage by exposing yourself to bright light in the morning and avoiding bright light in the evening. This helps signal to your body that it's time to wake up or wind down, respectively, aligning your internal clock with the destination's time zone.

Melatonin Supplementation:

Melatonin is a hormone that helps regulate the sleep-wake cycle. Taking melatonin supplements in the days leading up to travel can aid in adjusting your body's melatonin release to match the new time zone. Consult with a healthcare professional to determine the appropriate dosage and timing for your specific needs.

Sleep Hygiene:

Prioritize good sleep hygiene practices to optimize your sleep quality before departure. Establish a relaxing bedtime routine that includes activities such as reading a book, taking a warm bath, or practicing relaxation techniques. Create a sleep-friendly environment by ensuring your bedroom is cool, dark, and quiet, and consider using earplugs or an eye mask if necessary.

Avoid Stimulants and Sedatives:

In the days leading up to your trip, it's advisable to limit or avoid substances that can disrupt your sleep, such as caffeine and alcohol. Caffeine is a stimulant that can interfere with your ability to fall asleep, while alcohol can disrupt the quality of your sleep. Aim to cut back on these substances to promote better sleep and enhance your body's readiness for the time zone adjustment.

Maintain a Consistent Sleep Schedule:

Consistency is key when it comes to sleep. Try to maintain a consistent sleep schedule in the days leading up to your departure. Go to bed and wake up at the same time each day, even on weekends. This helps regulate your body's internal clock and prepares it for the upcoming time zone change.

Exercise Regularly:

Engaging in regular physical activity can improve your sleep quality and aid in adjusting to a new time zone. Incorporate exercise into your daily routine, but avoid intense workouts close to bedtime, as they can be stimulating and make it harder to fall asleep.

Nutrition and Hydration:

Pay attention to your nutrition and hydration leading up to your trip. Eat a balanced diet that includes foods rich in sleep-promoting nutrients, such as tryptophan, magnesium, and vitamin B6. Stay hydrated by drinking plenty of water throughout the day, but be mindful of fluid intake close to bedtime to avoid disruptive trips to the bathroom.

Tips for Optimizing Your Physical and Mental State Prior to Travel

Preparing for travel goes beyond just packing your bags and booking your tickets. It is equally important to ensure that you are in the best possible physical and mental state before embarking on your journey. By optimizing your well-being, you can enhance your travel experience, minimize the impact of jet lag, and increase your overall enjoyment. These are various tips and strategies for optimizing your physical and mental state prior to travel.

1. Get Sufficient Rest:

Before embarking on your trip, make sure to prioritize rest and get sufficient sleep. Fatigue can exacerbate the effects of jet lag and leave you feeling drained during your travels. Aim to establish a regular sleep schedule and create a relaxing bedtime routine to ensure you are well-rested before your departure.

2. Eat a Balanced Diet:

Maintaining a healthy diet is crucial for fueling your body and boosting your immune system before travel. Consume a balanced diet that includes fruits, vegetables, lean proteins, and whole grains. Avoid excessive consumption of processed foods, sugary snacks, and caffeinated beverages, as they can lead to energy crashes and disrupt your sleep patterns.

3. Stay Hydrated:

Proper hydration is essential for optimal functioning of the body, especially during travel. Drink plenty of water and minimize the intake of dehydrating beverages such as alcohol and caffeine. Carry a reusable water bottle with you to ensure you stay hydrated throughout your journey.

4. Exercise Regularly:

Engaging in regular physical activity before travel has numerous benefits. Exercise not only helps boost your overall fitness but also enhances your mood, reduces stress, and improves sleep quality. Incorporate a mix of cardio, strength training, and flexibility exercises into your routine to prepare your body for the physical demands of travel.

5. Manage Stress:

Travel can be exciting, but it can also be accompanied by stress and anxiety. Prioritize stress management techniques such as meditation, deep breathing exercises, yoga, or journaling. Engaging in activities that bring you joy and relaxation can help alleviate pre-travel stress and promote a positive mindset.

6. Boost Your Immune System:

Travel often exposes us to new environments and potential illness. Prior to your trip, take steps to boost your immune system. Ensure you are up to date on any necessary vaccinations, consume immune-boosting foods rich in vitamins and minerals, and consider taking supplements like vitamin C and zinc to support your immune function.

7. Plan and Organize:

Effective planning and organization can significantly reduce pre-travel stress. Create a checklist of essential items to pack, research your destination, and familiarize yourself with important information such as local customs, transportation options, and emergency contacts. This preparation will help you feel more confident and relaxed before you depart.

8. Take Care of Personal Responsibilities:

Before you leave, address any personal responsibilities or tasks that may cause undue stress during your trip. Pay bills, inform your bank of your travel plans, and make arrangements for the care of pets or plants. Clearing these responsibilities will allow you to focus on enjoying your journey without distractions.

9. Practice Mindfulness:

Cultivating mindfulness can enhance your travel experience by helping you stay present and appreciate each moment. Engage in mindfulness practices such as mindful breathing, observing your surroundings, or practicing gratitude. These techniques can help reduce anxiety, improve focus, and foster a deeper connection with your travel experiences.

10. Seek Support:

If you feel overwhelmed or anxious about your upcoming journey, do not hesitate to seek support from loved ones or professionals. Talking about your concerns and getting reassurance can provide valuable emotional support and help alleviate any pre-travel jitters.

Chapter 3

In-Flight Strategies for a Smooth Transition

Techniques for Managing Sleep, Hydration, and Nutrition During Flights

Long flights can often disrupt our sleep patterns, leave us feeling dehydrated, and make it challenging to maintain a balanced diet. However, with the right strategies and preparation, you can effectively manage these aspects and ensure a smoother transition to your destination. In this chapter, we will explore various techniques for managing sleep, hydration, and nutrition during flights, allowing you to arrive refreshed and ready to adjust to the new time zone.

1. Prioritize Sleep:

Getting quality sleep during a long flight can significantly impact your energy levels and minimize the effects of jet lag. Consider the following tips to optimize your sleep experience:

- Choose the Right Seat: Select a seat that allows for maximum comfort and minimizes disruptions. Window seats offer a place to lean against, while aisle seats provide easy access to stretch your legs.

- Wear Comfortable Clothing: Dress in loose-fitting, breathable attire that allows for ease of movement and promotes comfort during sleep.

- Use Travel Pillows and Blankets: Bring a travel pillow and a cozy blanket to enhance your sleeping environment and provide support for your neck and back.

Rise Above Jet Lag

- Block Out Noise and Light: Use earplugs, noise-canceling headphones, and an eye mask to create a quiet and dark environment that promotes better sleep.

- Set Your Watch to the Destination Time: Adjust your mindset by setting your watch to the local time of your destination. This helps you mentally align with the new time zone and facilitates better sleep.

- Follow Sleep Rituals: Incorporate pre-sleep rituals, such as reading a book, listening to calming music, or practicing relaxation techniques, to signal your body that it's time to wind down and prepare for sleep.

2. Stay Hydrated:

Airplane cabins are notorious for their dry air, which can lead to dehydration. Proper hydration is crucial for maintaining energy levels and overall well-being during the flight. Consider the following tips to stay adequately hydrated:

- Drink Plenty of Water: Regularly sip on water throughout the flight to replenish lost fluids. Consider bringing a reusable water bottle to ensure easy access to hydration.

- Limit Alcohol and Caffeine: Both alcohol and caffeinated beverages can contribute to dehydration. Minimize your consumption of these drinks or avoid them altogether during the flight.

- Moisturize Your Skin: Apply a hydrating facial mist and use a moisturizer to prevent your skin from drying out due to the cabin's dry air.

- Use Saline Nasal Spray: Nasal passages can become dry during the flight, leading to discomfort and congestion. Use a saline nasal spray to keep your nasal passages moist.

3. Optimize Nutrition:

Maintaining a balanced diet during a flight can be challenging due to limited food options and the temptation of unhealthy snacks. However, with some planning, you can make conscious choices to nourish your body. Consider the following tips to optimize your nutrition during the flight:

- Pack Healthy Snacks: Bring nutrient-rich snacks such as fresh fruits, granola bars, trail mix, or cut-up vegetables to keep you satisfied and energized throughout the flight.

- Choose Balanced Meal Options: When selecting in-flight meals, opt for options that include a balance of protein, carbohydrates, and vegetables. Avoid heavy, greasy meals that can leave you feeling sluggish.

- Avoid Excessive Salt and Sugar: Airline meals can sometimes be high in sodium and added sugars. Be mindful of your salt and sugar intake to prevent bloating and energy crashes.

- Hydrate with Water, Herbal Tea, or Infused Water: Instead of sugary beverages, opt for water, herbal tea, or infused water to stay hydrated and avoid unnecessary calories.

- Limit Processed Foods: Try to avoid or limit consumption of highly processed snacks and meals, as they are often low in nutrients and high in additives.

4. Incorporate Movement and Stretching:

Sitting for an extended period can lead to muscle stiffness and discomfort. Incorporating movement and stretching exercises during the flight can help improve circulation and reduce stiffness. Consider the following techniques:

- Take Regular Walks: Get up and walk around the cabin whenever it is safe to do so. This helps promote blood circulation and prevents stiffness.

- Perform In-Seat Exercises: Engage in simple exercises that can be done while seated, such as ankle rolls, leg lifts, shoulder rolls, and neck stretches. These movements help keep your muscles active and prevent stiffness.

5. Practice Mindfulness and Relaxation Techniques:

Flying can be stressful for some individuals. Incorporating mindfulness and relaxation techniques can help alleviate anxiety and promote a sense of calm during the flight. Consider the following practices:

- Deep Breathing: Practice deep breathing exercises to promote relaxation and reduce stress. Inhale deeply through your nose, hold for a few seconds, and exhale slowly through your mouth.

- Meditation or Guided Visualization: Use meditation or guided visualization techniques to calm your mind and focus on positive imagery.

- Listen to Relaxing Music or Audiobooks: Prepare a playlist of relaxing music or listen to audiobooks that promote tranquility and help you unwind.

Ways to Create a Comfortable Environment for Better Rest and Recovery

Creating a comfortable environment is crucial for promoting better rest and recovery. Whether it's your bedroom, a hotel room, or a temporary accommodation, certain factors can significantly impact the quality of your sleep. Let's see various ways to create a comfortable environment that promotes relaxation, enhances sleep quality, and supports your body's natural recovery processes.

1. Optimize Lighting:

Lighting plays a significant role in regulating our sleep-wake cycle. Consider the following tips to optimize lighting for better rest:

- Dim the Lights: As bedtime approaches, dim the lights in your bedroom to signal to your body that it's time to wind down. Avoid bright and harsh lights, as they can interfere with your body's production of melatonin, the hormone responsible for promoting sleep.

- Use Blackout Curtains or Eye Masks: Block out external sources of light using blackout curtains or wear an eye mask to create a dark environment conducive to sleep. This is particularly beneficial if you live in an area with streetlights or if you are traveling and facing unfamiliar light sources.

- Incorporate Warm Lighting: Instead of bright white lights, opt for warm, soft lighting in your bedroom. Consider using bedside lamps with warm-colored bulbs or installing dimmer switches to adjust the lighting intensity to your preference.

2. Set the Right Temperature:

Maintaining an optimal temperature in your sleep environment is essential for promoting better sleep. Consider the following tips to set the right temperature:

- Keep Your Bedroom Cool: The ideal temperature for sleep is typically between 60 to 67 degrees Fahrenheit (15 to 19 degrees Celsius). Adjust your thermostat or use fans or air conditioning to create a cool and comfortable sleep environment.

- Use Breathable Bedding: Choose bedding materials that are breathable and help regulate body temperature, such as cotton or bamboo sheets, and lightweight, breathable blankets or comforters.

- Layer Your Bedding: Opt for layering your bedding, so you can easily adjust the number of covers to maintain a comfortable temperature throughout the night.

3. Minimize Noise:

Noise can disrupt sleep and prevent you from entering into deep, restorative sleep cycles. Consider the following tips to minimize noise in your sleep environment:

- Use Earplugs or White Noise Machines: If you're sensitive to noise, consider using earplugs or white noise machines to drown out disruptive sounds and create a more peaceful environment for sleep.

- Soundproof Your Room: If external noise is a persistent issue, consider soundproofing your bedroom by using soundproof curtains, rugs, or installing soundproofing panels on walls.

4. Create a Clutter-Free Space:

A clutter-free environment can promote relaxation and a sense of calm. Consider the following tips to create a clutter-free space:

- Declutter Your Bedroom: Remove unnecessary items and keep surfaces clear of clutter. Create designated storage spaces for belongings to maintain an organized and serene atmosphere.

- Choose Soothing Colors: Select calming and soothing colors for your bedroom walls and decor. Soft neutrals, pastels, or cool tones can contribute to a relaxing atmosphere.

5. Invest in Comfortable Bedding and Furniture:

The quality of your mattress, pillows, and other furniture can significantly impact your comfort and sleep quality. Consider the following tips:

- Choose a Supportive Mattress: Invest in a mattress that provides adequate support and aligns with your personal comfort preferences. It's important to find a mattress that promotes proper spinal alignment and minimizes pressure points.

- Find the Right Pillows: Select pillows that offer proper neck and head support. There are various pillow options available, such as memory foam, down alternative, or cervical pillows. Experiment with different types to find the one that suits your needs best.

- Consider Ergonomic Furniture: If you have a dedicated workspace or reading area in your bedroom, choose ergonomic furniture that promotes good posture and reduces strain on your body.

Chapter 4

Time Zone Transition Techniques

Expert Strategies for Minimizing the Impact of Changing Time Zones

Changing time zones can disrupt our body's internal clock and lead to symptoms of jet lag, including fatigue, difficulty sleeping, and decreased cognitive function. However, with the right strategies, you can minimize the impact of time zone transitions and adjust more smoothly to your new destination. Let's see some expert techniques and strategies for navigating time zone transitions effectively.

1. Adjust Your Sleep Schedule Before Travel:

One of the key factors in minimizing the impact of time zone transitions is to gradually adjust your sleep schedule before your trip. Consider the following strategies:

- Shift Your Sleep and Wake Times: Gradually adjust your sleep and wake times in the days leading up to your trip. Shift them closer to the schedule of your destination's time zone to align your body with the new time.

- Use Light Exposure: Exposure to natural light or artificial light that mimics sunlight can help regulate your body's internal clock. Seek bright light in the morning to signal wakefulness and dim the lights in the evening to promote relaxation and prepare your body for sleep.

2. Stay Hydrated and Mindful of Nutrition:

Proper hydration and mindful nutrition play a crucial role in supporting your body's adjustment to a new time zone. Consider the following tips:

- Hydrate Before, During, and After the Flight: Drink plenty of water before, during, and after your flight to stay hydrated. Dehydration can exacerbate the symptoms of jet lag, so it's important to keep your body hydrated.

- Eat Light and Balanced Meals: Opt for light and balanced meals during your journey, focusing on whole foods, fruits, vegetables, and lean proteins. Avoid heavy, greasy, or processed foods that can disrupt digestion and impact sleep quality.

- Be Mindful of Caffeine and Alcohol Consumption: Caffeine and alcohol can affect sleep patterns and worsen jet lag symptoms. Limit your intake or avoid these substances close to bedtime to support a more restful sleep.

3. Adjust Your Routine Upon Arrival:

Once you reach your destination, making adjustments to your routine can help your body adapt to the new time zone. Consider the following techniques:

- Get on Local Time: Immediately adjust your activities, including meals, exercise, and sleep, to align with the local time zone. This helps your body sync with the new schedule more quickly.

- Seek Natural Light: Spend time outdoors and expose yourself to natural light during daylight hours. This can help reset your body's internal clock and promote alertness during the day.

- Avoid Napping for Extended Periods: While a short power nap can be beneficial, avoid napping for extended periods, as it can disrupt your nighttime sleep. Try to stay awake until the local bedtime to facilitate a smoother transition.

4. Utilize Strategic Light Exposure:

Light exposure can be a powerful tool in adjusting to a new time zone. Consider the following strategies:

- Seek Morning Light: Expose yourself to natural light or bright light in the morning, as it helps signal wakefulness and reset your internal clock.

- Minimize Evening Light: In the evening, reduce your exposure to bright lights, especially blue light emitted by electronic devices, as it can suppress the production of melatonin and interfere with sleep.

- Use Light Therapy: If necessary, consider using light therapy devices or special lightboxes that simulate daylight to regulate your circadian rhythm and support adjustment to a new time zone.

5. Adopt Sleep-Enhancing Practices:

Establishing a sleep-enhancing routine can significantly improve sleep quality and aid in adjusting to a new time zone. Consider the following practices:

- Create a Relaxing Bedtime Routine: Develop a pre-sleep routine that helps signal to your body that it's time to wind down. This may include

activities like reading a book, taking a warm bath, or practicing relaxation techniques such as meditation or deep breathing exercises.

- Optimize Your Sleep Environment: Ensure your sleep environment is conducive to quality rest. This includes maintaining a cool temperature, minimizing noise, using comfortable bedding and pillows, and creating a dark and quiet space.

- Consider Sleep Aids: In consultation with a healthcare professional, you may explore the use of sleep aids such as melatonin supplements or herbal remedies to support sleep quality during the time zone transition. However, it's important to use these aids responsibly and according to the recommended dosage.

Advice on When and How to Adjust Sleep and Meal Times to Facilitate Adaptation

One of the key challenges in overcoming jet lag is adjusting your sleep and meal times to align with your new time zone. By strategically timing your activities, you can help your body adapt more quickly to the local schedule and minimize the symptoms of jet lag.

1. Assessing the Time Difference:

Before you embark on your journey, it's crucial to understand the time difference between your departure and arrival destinations. Take note of the number of time zones you will be crossing and the direction of travel (eastward or westward). This information will serve as a foundation for planning your sleep and meal adjustments.

2. Gradual Adjustments:

Adjusting your sleep and meal times gradually is a key strategy for facilitating adaptation to a new time zone. Rather than making sudden shifts, follow these recommendations:

- Start Shifting Prior to Departure: Begin gradually shifting your sleep and meal times a few days before your trip. If you're traveling east, try advancing your sleep and meal times by 30 minutes to an hour each day. If you're traveling west, delay them by the same increments.

- Plan in Sync with Your Destination: Use the time zone of your destination as a guide for adjusting your activities. Begin aligning your sleep and meal times with the local schedule, taking into account the time you will arrive.

- Allow Ample Time for Adjustment: Depending on the number of time zones you are crossing, give yourself several days to adjust your sleep and meal times gradually. This allows your body to adapt more smoothly and reduces the severity of jet lag symptoms.

3. Syncing Sleep and Light Exposure:

Light exposure plays a significant role in regulating your body's internal clock. By syncing your sleep and light exposure, you can aid in the adaptation process. Consider the following tips:

- Seek Morning Light: Expose yourself to natural light or bright light in the morning at your destination. This helps signal wakefulness to your body and encourages the synchronization of your internal clock.

- Minimize Evening Light: In the evening, limit your exposure to bright lights, especially blue light emitted by electronic devices. Blue light suppresses melatonin production and can interfere with your ability to fall asleep and adjust to the local schedule.

- Utilize Light Therapy: If necessary, consider using light therapy devices or special lightboxes designed to mimic natural light. These can help regulate your circadian rhythm and facilitate adaptation to a new time zone.

4. Adjusting Meal Times:

Meal times can also influence your body's internal clock. Here are some tips for adjusting your meal times effectively:

Rise Above Jet Lag

- Time Your Meals with Local Schedule: Once you arrive at your destination, begin aligning your meal times with the local schedule. This helps synchronize your digestive system and supports your body's adaptation to the new time zone.

- Consider Fasting: Some individuals find that implementing a short-term fasting approach can help adjust their meal times more quickly. This involves restricting food intake for a set period before gradually reintroducing meals according to the local schedule.

- Stay Hydrated: While adjusting your meal times, remember to stay hydrated. Drink plenty of water throughout the day to maintain hydration levels and support your overall well-being.

5. Sleep and Meal Strategies During Transit:

When traveling long distances, particularly on flights that span several time zones, it's essential to employ strategies that promote restful sleep and appropriate meal timing. Consider the following suggestions:

- Adjust Sleep on Long Flights: If your flight aligns with your destination's nighttime, aim to get some sleep during the journey. Use sleep aids, eye masks, noise-canceling headphones, and comfortable travel pillows to create a conducive sleep environment.

- Optimize Nutrition During Travel: Plan your meals and snacks on long flights according to the destination's meal times. Choose nourishing foods that support your energy levels and avoid heavy meals that can disrupt your sleep or digestion.

Chapter 5

Sleep Optimization for Jet Lag Recovery

Establishing Healthy Sleep Habits to Enhance Recovery and Combat Jet Lag

Quality sleep is essential for overcoming jet lag and promoting a speedy recovery. In this chapter, we will delve into the importance of establishing healthy sleep habits to optimize your sleep and combat jet lag. By implementing these strategies, you can enhance your recovery, adjust to the new time zone more effectively, and experience a smoother transition.

1. Prioritize Consistency:

Consistency is key when it comes to healthy sleep habits. Aim to maintain a regular sleep schedule, even during travel. Here are some tips to help you prioritize consistency:

- Set a Sleep Schedule: Determine the ideal bedtime and wake-up time based on the local time zone. Stick to this schedule as closely as possible, even on weekends or during non-travel days.

- Avoid Napping: While it may be tempting to take a nap to combat fatigue, try to resist the urge. Napping can disrupt your sleep-wake cycle and make it harder to adjust to the new time zone.

2. Create a Sleep-Friendly Environment:

Your sleep environment plays a significant role in promoting quality rest. Consider the following factors to create a sleep-friendly environment:

- Optimize Lighting: Make your sleep environment as dark as possible. Use blackout curtains or eye masks to block out light that can interfere with sleep.

- Control Noise Levels: Minimize noise disruptions by using earplugs or white noise machines. These can help drown out external noises and create a more peaceful sleep environment.

- Regulate Temperature: Keep the room temperature cool and comfortable. Adjust the thermostat or use fans or blankets to achieve an optimal sleep temperature.

- Choose Comfortable Bedding: Select a comfortable mattress, pillows, and bedding that provide adequate support and ensure a restful sleep.

3. Establish a Relaxing Bedtime Routine:

A relaxing bedtime routine can signal to your body that it's time to wind down and prepare for sleep. Consider incorporating the following practices into your routine:

- Disconnect from Screens: Avoid electronic devices, such as smartphones or tablets, before bed. The blue light emitted by these devices can interfere with the production of melatonin, a hormone that regulates sleep.

- Engage in Relaxation Techniques: Practice relaxation techniques such as deep breathing exercises, progressive muscle relaxation, or meditation to calm your mind and body before sleep.

- Read or Listen to Soothing Content: Engage in a relaxing activity, such as reading a book or listening to calming music or podcasts, to help you unwind before bed.

- Take a Warm Bath: A warm bath or shower before bed can promote relaxation and prepare your body for sleep.

4. Manage Stress and Anxiety:

Stress and anxiety can significantly impact your sleep quality and exacerbate jet lag symptoms. Implement the following strategies to manage stress and promote better sleep:

- Practice Stress Reduction Techniques: Explore stress reduction techniques such as mindfulness, yoga, or journaling. These practices can help you relax, clear your mind, and alleviate stress before bed.

- Seek Support: If stress or anxiety is persistent and impacting your sleep, consider seeking support from a mental health professional who can provide guidance and tools for stress management.

5. Embrace Healthy Sleep Habits:

In addition to the above strategies, incorporating healthy sleep habits into your daily routine can further enhance your sleep quality and recovery from jet lag. Consider the following tips:

- Engage in Regular Physical Activity: Regular exercise can improve sleep quality and help regulate your body's internal clock. However, avoid intense exercise close to bedtime, as it can stimulate your body and make it harder to fall asleep.

- Limit Caffeine and Alcohol Intake: Caffeine and alcohol can disrupt your sleep patterns and exacerbate jet lag symptoms. Limit your consumption of these substances, especially in the hours leading up to bedtime.

- Create a Comfortable Sleep Environment: Ensure that your sleep environment is comfortable, clean, and conducive to quality sleep. Keep your bedroom clutter-free, maintain a cool temperature, and invest in comfortable bedding.

Sleep Hygiene Practices and Relaxation Techniques for Improved Sleep Quality

Sleep hygiene practices and relaxation techniques play a vital role in promoting optimal sleep quality. Let's see various strategies and habits that can help improve your sleep hygiene and enhance the overall quality of your sleep. By implementing these practices and techniques, you can create a conducive environment for restful sleep and experience the many benefits of a good night's rest.

1. Establish a Consistent Sleep Schedule:

Maintaining a regular sleep schedule is key to improving sleep quality. Consider the following tips:

- Set a Fixed Bedtime and Wake-Up Time: Establish a consistent sleep routine by going to bed and waking up at the same time each day, even on weekends.

- Avoid Oversleeping: Resist the temptation to oversleep, as it can disrupt your sleep-wake cycle and lead to grogginess and fatigue.

2. Create a Relaxing Bedtime Routine:

A relaxing bedtime routine can signal to your body that it's time to unwind and prepare for sleep. Here are some practices to incorporate into your routine:

- Establish a Wind-Down Period: Allocate time before bed to relax and engage in calming activities, such as reading, listening to soothing music, or taking a warm bath.

- Limit Screen Time: Avoid electronic devices, such as smartphones, tablets, or laptops, before bed as the blue light emitted by these devices can interfere with the production of melatonin, a hormone that regulates sleep.

- Practice Relaxation Techniques: Explore relaxation techniques such as deep breathing exercises, progressive muscle relaxation, or guided imagery to help calm your mind and prepare your body for sleep.

3. Create a Sleep-Friendly Environment:

Your sleep environment can significantly impact your sleep quality. Consider the following tips:

- Optimize Lighting: Make your bedroom as dark as possible by using blackout curtains or an eye mask to block out external light sources.

- Control Noise Levels: Minimize noise disruptions by using earplugs or a white noise machine to create a peaceful sleep environment.

- Regulate Temperature: Maintain a comfortable temperature in your bedroom that promotes restful sleep. Adjust the thermostat or use blankets and fans as needed.

- Choose Comfortable Bedding: Select a comfortable mattress, pillows, and bedding that provide adequate support and promote a comfortable sleep posture.

4. Practice Healthy Lifestyle Habits:

Certain lifestyle habits can impact your sleep quality. Consider the following tips:

- Regular Exercise: Engage in regular physical activity, but avoid exercising too close to bedtime as it can energize your body and make it harder to fall asleep.

- Balanced Diet: Adopt a balanced diet that includes sleep-supportive nutrients such as magnesium, tryptophan, and vitamins B6 and C. Avoid heavy meals close to bedtime that can disrupt digestion and interfere with sleep.

- Limit Stimulants: Reduce your intake of stimulants such as caffeine and nicotine, especially in the hours leading up to bedtime, as they can interfere with sleep.

5. Manage Stress and Anxiety:

Stress and anxiety can significantly impact sleep quality. Consider the following tips for stress management:

- Practice Stress-Relief Techniques: Explore stress-relief techniques such as meditation, mindfulness, yoga, or journaling to calm your mind and reduce stress before bed.

- Create a Relaxing Environment: Make your bedroom a peaceful and stress-free space by decluttering and creating a serene ambiance that promotes relaxation.

Chapter 6

Nutrition and Hydration for Energy and Vitality

Guidance on Nourishing Foods and Hydration Practices to Support Energy Levels

Proper nutrition and hydration play a crucial role in maintaining optimal energy levels and overall vitality. In this chapter, we will explore the importance of nourishing foods and hydration practices for sustaining energy throughout the day. By incorporating healthy eating habits and maintaining proper hydration, you can fuel your body with the nutrients it needs to thrive. Let's dive into the world of nutrition and discover how to boost your energy and vitality through smart food choices and hydration practices.

1. Understanding the Role of Nutrients:

Before we delve into specific foods, it's important to understand the role of nutrients in providing energy and supporting overall well-being. Consider the following key nutrients:

- Carbohydrates: Carbohydrates are the body's primary source of energy. Choose complex carbohydrates like whole grains, fruits, and vegetables, as they provide sustained energy release.

- Proteins: Proteins are essential for tissue repair and maintenance. Opt for lean sources such as poultry, fish, legumes, and tofu to support muscle health and energy production.

- Healthy Fats: Incorporate healthy fats from sources like nuts, seeds, avocados, and olive oil. These fats provide a slow and steady release of energy and support brain function.

- Vitamins and Minerals: Ensure you consume a variety of fruits, vegetables, and whole foods to obtain essential vitamins and minerals that contribute to overall energy production and vitality.

2. Energizing Foods for Sustained Energy:

Choose nutrient-dense foods that provide a steady supply of energy throughout the day. Consider the following:

- Whole Grains: Opt for whole grains like quinoa, brown rice, and oats, which are rich in complex carbohydrates and fiber for long-lasting energy.

- Fruits and Vegetables: Incorporate a colorful array of fruits and vegetables to provide essential vitamins, minerals, and antioxidants that support energy production.

- Lean Proteins: Include lean proteins such as chicken, turkey, fish, beans, and lentils, which provide a steady source of amino acids for sustained energy and muscle repair.

- Healthy Fats: Incorporate sources of healthy fats like nuts, seeds, avocados, and olive oil to provide sustained energy and support brain health.

- Hydration: Stay properly hydrated by drinking an adequate amount of water throughout the day. Dehydration can cause fatigue and impair cognitive function, so aim to drink water regularly.

3. Timing and Meal Frequency:

In addition to making wise food choices, consider the timing of your meals and snacks to sustain energy levels:

- Regular Meals: Aim for three balanced meals per day to provide a consistent source of energy. Include a combination of carbohydrates, proteins, and healthy fats in each meal.

- Smart Snacking: Incorporate healthy snacks between meals to maintain energy levels and prevent energy crashes. Choose nutrient-dense options like fruits, nuts, yogurt, or whole-grain crackers.

- Balanced Macros: Ensure that each meal and snack contains a balance of carbohydrates, proteins, and fats for sustained energy release and satiety.

4. Hydration Strategies for Energy:

Proper hydration is essential for energy and vitality. Consider the following hydration strategies:

- Water Intake: Drink an adequate amount of water throughout the day. Aim for at least eight glasses of water, or more depending on your activity level and climate.

- Electrolyte Balance: Replenish electrolytes lost through sweat by incorporating electrolyte-rich beverages or consuming foods like coconut water, fruits, and vegetables.

- Limit Caffeine and Alcohol: While small amounts of caffeine can provide a temporary energy boost, excessive caffeine and alcohol consumption can disrupt sleep patterns and lead to energy crashes.

5. Tailoring Nutrition for Individual Needs:

Every individual's nutritional needs may vary based on factors like age, sex, activity level, and health conditions. Consult with a registered dietitian or nutritionist to personalize your nutrition plan and ensure you're meeting your specific energy requirements.

Recommendations for Meals and Snacks that Aid in Reducing Jet Lag Symptoms

Let's dive into the world of jet lag nutrition and discover how to nourish your body for a smoother transition.

1. Balanced Meals for Time Zone Adaptation:

When it comes to meals, opting for balanced and nutritious options can contribute to a more seamless adjustment to a new time zone. Consider the following recommendations:

- Include a mix of macronutrients: Aim to incorporate a balance of carbohydrates, proteins, and healthy fats in your meals. This combination provides sustained energy and helps regulate your body's internal clock.

- Focus on whole foods: Choose whole, unprocessed foods whenever possible. They are rich in essential nutrients and support overall well-being.

- Prioritize lean proteins: Include lean sources of protein such as poultry, fish, tofu, and legumes.

Protein helps regulate sleep-wake cycles and promotes alertness during the day.

- Incorporate complex carbohydrates: Opt for complex carbohydrates like whole grains, fruits, and vegetables. They provide a steady release of energy and aid in maintaining stable blood sugar levels.

- Include healthy fats: Incorporate sources of healthy fats such as avocados, nuts, seeds, and olive oil. These fats provide sustained energy and support brain function.

2. Meal Timing and Frequency:

The timing and frequency of meals can also play a role in minimizing jet lag symptoms. Consider the following recommendations:

- Adjust meal times gradually: Before traveling, gradually shift your meal times closer to your destination's time zone. This helps your body adjust to the new schedule in advance.

- Lighter meals before sleep: As bedtime approaches, opt for lighter meals that are easier to digest. This can help promote better sleep quality and minimize digestive discomfort.

- Regular meal intervals: Aim for regular meal intervals throughout the day to keep your body nourished and energized. Avoid prolonged periods without food to prevent energy crashes.

3. Snacks for Sustained Energy:

In addition to meals, strategically chosen snacks can provide sustained energy and help alleviate jet lag symptoms. Consider the following recommendations:

- Nutrient-dense snacks: Choose snacks that are rich in nutrients and provide a combination of carbohydrates, proteins, and healthy fats. This combination helps maintain stable energy levels.

- Portable options: Opt for portable snacks that are easy to pack and consume during travel. Examples include trail mix, energy bars, fruits, and yogurt cups.

- Hydrating snacks: Include snacks with high water content, such as cucumber slices, watermelon, or celery sticks, to stay hydrated during your journey.

- Avoid sugary snacks: While sugary snacks may provide a temporary energy boost, they can lead to energy crashes and disrupt your sleep-wake cycles.

4. Hydration for Jet Lag Relief:

Proper hydration is crucial for combating jet lag symptoms. Consider the following hydration recommendations:

- Drink water regularly: Stay hydrated by drinking water regularly throughout your journey. Dehydration can exacerbate jet lag symptoms and lead to fatigue.

- Limit caffeine and alcohol: While caffeine can provide a temporary energy boost, excessive consumption can disrupt sleep patterns. Similarly, alcohol can impair sleep quality and exacerbate jet lag symptoms.

- Hydrating foods: Include hydrating foods in your diet, such as cucumbers, watermelon, oranges, and leafy greens. These foods can contribute to your overall hydration levels.

Chapter 7

Active Strategies for Circadian Rhythm Adjustment

Circadian rhythms play a crucial role in regulating our sleep-wake cycles and overall well-being. When traveling across time zones or experiencing disruptions to our daily routines, our circadian rhythms can become imbalanced, leading to difficulties in adjusting to new sleep patterns. However, by incorporating active strategies into our daily lives, we can help regulate our circadian rhythms, promote restful sleep, and enhance overall sleep quality. In this chapter, we will explore various techniques, including physical activity, light exposure, and mindful practices, that can aid in circadian rhythm adjustment. Let's dive into the world of active strategies and discover how they can contribute to better sleep and well-being.

1. The Role of Physical Activity:

Physical activity has been shown to have a positive impact on sleep and circadian rhythm regulation. Consider the following recommendations:

- Regular exercise: Engage in regular physical exercise to promote a healthy sleep-wake cycle. Aim for at least 150 minutes of moderate-intensity aerobic activity or 75 minutes of vigorous-intensity activity each week.

- Timing of exercise: Try to schedule your exercise sessions earlier in the day, as exercising close to bedtime may interfere with sleep. However, individual preferences may vary, so listen to your body and adjust accordingly.

- Outdoor activities: Whenever possible, engage in outdoor activities. Natural light exposure during physical activity can help regulate circadian rhythms and enhance sleep quality.

- Mind-body exercises: Incorporate mind-body exercises such as yoga, tai chi, or qigong into your routine. These practices combine physical movement with mindful awareness, promoting relaxation and stress reduction.

2. Light Exposure and Circadian Rhythm Regulation:

Light exposure plays a crucial role in regulating our circadian rhythms. Consider the following recommendations:

- Morning light exposure: Expose yourself to natural sunlight or bright indoor light in the morning to signal wakefulness and reset your internal clock. Open curtains or go outside for a walk to maximize light exposure.

- Dim lighting in the evening: Create a dim and relaxing environment in the evening to signal the body's preparation for sleep. Avoid bright screens, such as smartphones and tablets, at least one hour before bedtime, as the blue light emitted can suppress the production of melatonin, a hormone that helps regulate sleep.

- Light therapy: In cases where natural light exposure is limited, consider using light therapy devices that mimic natural sunlight. These devices can help regulate circadian rhythms and promote better sleep quality.

3. Mindful Practices for Sleep and Relaxation:

Mindfulness practices can be effective tools for managing stress, promoting relaxation, and improving sleep. Consider the following recommendations:

- Meditation and deep breathing exercises: Incorporate regular meditation or deep breathing exercises into your daily routine. These practices can help calm the mind, reduce stress, and prepare the body for restful sleep.

- Progressive muscle relaxation: Practice progressive muscle relaxation techniques, where you systematically tense and relax different muscle groups in your body. This practice promotes physical relaxation and can aid in falling asleep more easily.

- Sleep hygiene rituals: Establish a bedtime routine that includes activities to signal your body that it's time to wind down and prepare for sleep. This can include activities such as reading a book, taking a warm bath, or practicing gentle stretching.

- Stress management techniques: Find effective stress management techniques that work for you, such as journaling, engaging in creative activities, or seeking support from a therapist or counselor. By managing stress, you can create a more conducive environment for quality sleep.

Techniques for Syncing Your Body's Internal Clock with the New Time Zone

1. Gradual Time Adjustment:

One effective technique for syncing your body's internal clock with the new time zone is to gradually adjust your sleep and wake times before your trip. Consider the following recommendations:

- Shifting sleep and wake times: Start adjusting your sleep and wake times a few days before your departure. Gradually shift them closer to the local time of your destination. For example, if you're traveling eastward, try going to bed and waking up an hour earlier each day leading up to your trip.

- Light exposure: Use natural light exposure to help regulate your circadian rhythm. Get plenty of sunlight in the morning at your destination to signal wakefulness, and avoid bright light in the evening to promote the release of melatonin, a hormone that regulates sleep.

- Melatonin supplementation: Consult with your healthcare provider about the potential benefits of melatonin supplementation. Melatonin is a hormone that helps regulate sleep-wake cycles, and taking it at the appropriate time can aid in adjusting to a new time zone.

2. Strategic Napping:

Napping strategically can help you manage fatigue and adjust to the new time zone. Consider the following tips:

- Short and timed naps: Take short, timed naps during the day to combat daytime sleepiness. Limit your nap duration to 20-30 minutes to avoid disrupting your nighttime sleep.

- Avoid long naps: Avoid long naps that can interfere with your ability to fall asleep at night. Long naps may also make it harder for your body to adjust to the new time zone.

- Optimal nap timing: Time your naps strategically based on your travel itinerary and the local time zone. Taking a nap during the mid-afternoon, around 2-3 p.m., can provide a quick energy boost without disrupting your nighttime sleep.

3. Light Therapy:

Light therapy involves exposing yourself to specific wavelengths of light to regulate your circadian rhythm. Consider the following recommendations:

Rise Above Jet Lag

- Morning light exposure: Expose yourself to bright light, preferably natural sunlight, in the morning at your destination. This helps signal wakefulness and resets your internal clock.

- Light-blocking eyewear: If you're traveling westward and need to adjust to an earlier bedtime, consider using light-blocking eyewear in the evening. These glasses filter out blue light, which can suppress melatonin production and interfere with your ability to fall asleep.

- Light boxes: Light boxes emit bright, artificial light that mimics natural sunlight. Using a light box in the morning at your destination can help reset your circadian rhythm and promote alertness.

4. Controlled Caffeine and Alcohol Consumption:

Caffeine and alcohol can disrupt your sleep-wake cycle and interfere with circadian rhythm adjustment. Consider the following guidelines:

- Limit caffeine intake: If you're sensitive to caffeine, avoid consuming it in the afternoon and evening. Caffeine can delay sleep onset and disrupt your sleep quality.

- Moderate alcohol consumption: While it may be tempting to have a nightcap to help you relax, alcohol can disrupt your sleep patterns and contribute to jet lag symptoms. Limit alcohol consumption, especially close to bedtime.

- Hydration: Stay hydrated by drinking plenty of water. Dehydration can exacerbate the symptoms of jet lag, so make sure to drink water throughout your journey.

Chapter 8

Natural Remedies and Supplements for Jet Lag Relief

We will be talking about a range of natural remedies and supplements that have shown promise in providing jet lag relief. It's important to note that these remedies and supplements should be used in conjunction with other strategies and lifestyle adjustments for optimal results.

1. Melatonin:

Melatonin is a hormone naturally produced by the body that regulates sleep-wake cycles. It is available as a supplement and has been widely studied for its potential in alleviating jet lag symptoms. Consider the following:

- Timing and dosage: Take melatonin supplements close to the desired bedtime at your destination. Start with a low dose (around 0.5 to 3 mg) and adjust as needed.

- Consult a healthcare professional: Before using melatonin supplements, consult with a healthcare professional, especially if you have any underlying medical conditions or are taking other medications.

2. Herbal Remedies:

Certain herbs have been used for centuries to promote relaxation, improve sleep quality, and reduce fatigue. Here are a few herbal remedies that may assist in jet lag relief:

- Valerian root: Valerian root is known for its calming properties and can help promote relaxation and better sleep. It is available in various forms, including capsules, tea, and tinctures.

- Chamomile: Chamomile is a popular herbal remedy for its soothing effects. Drinking chamomile tea before bedtime may help relax the body and support better sleep.

- Passionflower: Passionflower has been used as a natural sedative and relaxant. It may help reduce anxiety and promote better sleep quality.

3. Adaptogenic Herbs:

Adaptogenic herbs are known for their ability to support the body's stress response and promote overall well-being. These herbs may assist in combating the physical and mental stress associated with jet lag. Consider the following adaptogenic herbs:

- Ashwagandha: Ashwagandha is an adaptogenic herb that may help reduce stress, improve sleep quality, and enhance overall energy levels.

- Rhodiola rosea: Rhodiola rosea is known for its energizing properties and may help combat fatigue and increase mental clarity.

- Ginseng: Ginseng is an adaptogenic herb that may enhance energy levels, improve focus, and reduce stress.

4. Essential Oils:

Essential oils have been used for their therapeutic properties, including relaxation and sleep support. Consider the following essential oils for jet lag relief:

- Lavender: Lavender essential oil is known for its calming and soothing effects. Diffuse lavender oil in your hotel room or add a few drops to a bath before bedtime to promote relaxation.

- Peppermint: Peppermint essential oil is invigorating and can help improve focus and energy levels. Diffuse peppermint oil or inhale it for a quick pick-me-up during the day.

- Eucalyptus: Eucalyptus essential oil has a refreshing aroma that can help clear the mind and enhance alertness. Use it in a diffuser or as a topical rub to support mental clarity.

5. Vitamin B Complex:

B vitamins play a crucial role in energy production and the functioning of the nervous system. A vitamin B complex supplement may help support energy levels and reduce fatigue associated with jet lag.

6. Hydration and Electrolyte Balance:

Maintaining hydration and electrolyte balance is important for overall well-being and can help alleviate jet lag symptoms. Consider the following:

- Drink plenty of water: Stay hydrated by drinking water throughout your journey.

 Avoid excessive caffeine and alcohol, as they can contribute to dehydration.

- Electrolyte-rich beverages: Consider hydrating with electrolyte-rich beverages such as coconut water or sports drinks to replenish essential minerals lost during travel.

7. Magnesium:

Magnesium is a mineral that plays a role in muscle relaxation, sleep regulation, and stress reduction. Taking a magnesium supplement or incorporating magnesium-rich foods into your diet may promote relaxation and better sleep.

8. Anti-Inflammatory Foods:

Inflammation can contribute to feelings of fatigue and discomfort. Consuming anti-inflammatory foods may help reduce inflammation and support overall well-being. Include the following in your diet:

- Fatty fish: Fish rich in omega-3 fatty acids, such as salmon and sardines, have anti-inflammatory properties.

- Dark leafy greens: Incorporate vegetables like spinach, kale, and Swiss chard, which are packed with antioxidants and anti-inflammatory compounds.

- Turmeric: Turmeric contains curcumin, a potent anti-inflammatory compound. Use turmeric in cooking or consider taking a curcumin supplement.

9. Herbal Teas:

Herbal teas can provide comfort and relaxation, making them a soothing option during travel. Consider the following herbal teas for jet lag relief:

- Peppermint tea: Peppermint tea can help soothe digestion and ease discomfort associated with travel.

- Ginger tea: Ginger tea can aid in digestion and reduce feelings of nausea, which may be experienced during jet lag.

- Lemon balm tea: Lemon balm tea has calming properties and can help promote relaxation and better sleep.

10. Stress-Reduction Techniques:

Managing stress is essential for jet lag relief. Incorporate stress-reduction techniques into your travel routine, such as:

- Meditation and deep breathing exercises: Practice mindfulness and deep breathing to promote relaxation and reduce stress.

- Yoga or stretching: Engage in gentle yoga poses or stretching exercises to release tension and promote relaxation.

Chapter 9

Productivity and Performance Optimization

By implementing these techniques, you can enhance your focus, boost cognitive function, and maximize your performance, allowing you to make the most of your time, whether for work or leisure.

1. Understanding the Impact of Jet Lag on Productivity:

Before delving into strategies for productivity optimization, it's crucial to understand how jet lag affects our cognitive abilities and performance. Consider the following:

- Disrupted sleep patterns: Jet lag can result in fragmented and inadequate sleep, leading to reduced alertness, decreased concentration, and impaired cognitive function.

- Fatigue and lethargy: The physical and mental fatigue associated with jet lag can hinder productivity, making it challenging to sustain focus and maintain high performance.

- Disrupted circadian rhythm: Jet lag disrupts our body's natural circadian rhythm, which regulates our sleep-wake cycle. This disruption can lead to decreased productivity and difficulty in adjusting to a new time zone.

2. Sleep Optimization for Enhanced Productivity:

Quality sleep is essential for optimal cognitive function and productivity. Implement the following strategies to optimize your sleep and enhance productivity:

- Establish a consistent sleep schedule: Set a regular sleep routine, even while traveling. Go to bed and wake up at the same time each day to train your body for a consistent sleep-wake cycle.

- Create a sleep-friendly environment: Ensure your sleep environment is conducive to restful sleep. Optimize lighting, temperature, and noise levels to create a calm and comfortable atmosphere.

- Practice relaxation techniques: Incorporate relaxation techniques before bedtime, such as deep breathing exercises, meditation, or gentle stretching, to promote relaxation and prepare your mind for sleep.

- Minimize exposure to electronic devices: The blue light emitted by electronic devices can interfere with your sleep. Limit screen time before bed or use blue light filters on your devices.

3. Nutrition for Cognitive Function and Energy:

Proper nutrition plays a vital role in maintaining cognitive function and sustaining energy levels. Consider the following nutritional strategies for enhanced productivity:

- Balanced meals: Consume well-balanced meals that include a combination of protein, complex carbohydrates, and healthy fats to provide sustained energy throughout the day.

- Brain-boosting foods: Incorporate foods rich in antioxidants, omega-3 fatty acids, and vitamins B, C, and E. Examples include blueberries, salmon, avocados, nuts, and leafy greens.

- Stay hydrated: Dehydration can lead to fatigue and decreased cognitive function. Drink plenty of water throughout the day to stay hydrated and maintain optimal brain function.

- Limit caffeine intake: While caffeine can temporarily enhance alertness, excessive consumption can disrupt sleep and lead to energy crashes. Moderation is key.

4. Time Management and Prioritization:

Efficient time management and prioritization are essential for maintaining productivity and maximizing performance. Consider the following strategies:

- Create a daily schedule: Plan your day in advance, allocating specific time slots for important tasks and commitments. This helps you stay organized and focused.

- Set realistic goals: Break larger tasks into smaller, manageable goals. Prioritize tasks based on urgency and importance to ensure efficient use of your time and resources.

- Utilize productivity tools: Explore productivity apps, task management tools, and time-tracking techniques to streamline your workflow and boost efficiency.

- Take strategic breaks: Incorporate short breaks into your work schedule to recharge and prevent mental fatigue. Use these breaks to stretch, take a walk, or practice relaxation techniques.

5. Cognitive Enhancement Techniques:

To optimize your cognitive function and mental acuity, consider implementing the following techniques:

- Mental exercises: Engage in activities that stimulate your brain, such as puzzles, brain teasers, or learning new skills. These exercises promote cognitive flexibility and enhance mental sharpness.

- Mindfulness and meditation: Practice mindfulness and meditation to improve focus, reduce stress, and enhance cognitive performance.

- Physical activity: Regular exercise improves blood flow to the brain, enhances cognitive function, and boosts overall productivity. Incorporate physical activity into your daily routine, even while traveling.

- Adequate rest and recovery: Allow yourself sufficient downtime for rest and recovery. Overworking and pushing yourself too hard can lead to burnout and decreased productivity in the long run.

Tips for Managing Work or Personal Commitments during Travel and Recovery

Traveling can sometimes coincide with work or personal commitments that cannot be postponed. Balancing these commitments while also allowing for recovery from jet lag can be challenging. By implementing these techniques, you can maintain productivity, fulfill your responsibilities, and ensure a smooth transition back to your regular routine.

1. Prioritize and Plan Ahead:

- Assess your commitments: Evaluate your work or personal commitments and identify the most critical tasks that require immediate attention.

- Plan your schedule: Create a detailed schedule that outlines your commitments, deadlines, and important meetings or events during your travel and recovery period.

- Delegate when possible: Delegate tasks that can be handled by colleagues, assistants, or family members to alleviate some of the workload.

- Set realistic expectations: Communicate your availability and manage expectations with colleagues, clients, or family members regarding response times and deliverables.

2. Effective Communication:

- Notify relevant parties: Inform colleagues, clients, or collaborators about your travel plans and availability. Provide them with alternative contact information or emergency protocols, if necessary.

- Utilize communication tools: Make use of technology and communication tools such as email, instant messaging, or video conferencing to stay connected and maintain open lines of communication.

- Set boundaries: Establish boundaries and communicate your availability during specific times of the day or week to ensure uninterrupted focus and rest.

3. Time Management:

- Prioritize important tasks: Identify the most important tasks or projects and allocate dedicated time to focus on them during your travel and recovery period.

- Break tasks into manageable chunks: Divide larger tasks into smaller, more manageable sub-tasks to make them less overwhelming and more achievable.

- Time blocking: Schedule specific time blocks for work-related activities, allowing for breaks and rest periods to prevent mental fatigue.

- Avoid multitasking: Focus on one task at a time to maintain concentration and produce higher-quality work.

4. Optimize Work Efficiency:

- Create a conducive work environment: Set up a designated workspace in your travel accommodation or hotel room that is comfortable, organized, and free from distractions.

- Minimize disruptions: Inform others around you about your work commitments and request uninterrupted time to focus on important tasks.

- Use productivity tools: Utilize digital productivity tools, project management software, or task management apps to streamline workflows and stay organized.

- Practice effective time management techniques: Prioritize important tasks, utilize time-blocking techniques, and leverage the Pomodoro technique (working in focused bursts with short breaks) to maximize productivity.

5. Self-Care and Recovery:

- Set aside dedicated recovery time: Allocate specific periods during your travel or upon return to focus on rest, relaxation, and jet lag recovery.

- Practice self-care rituals: Incorporate self-care activities into your routine, such as meditation, deep breathing exercises, gentle stretches, or journaling, to manage stress and promote well-being.

- Maintain a healthy lifestyle: Prioritize sleep, eat nutritious meals, stay hydrated, and engage in regular physical activity to support your energy levels and overall well-being.

- Delegate non-essential tasks: Identify tasks that can be delegated or postponed until after your recovery period to allow for adequate rest and recuperation.

Chapter 10

Long-Term Jet Lag Prevention and Management

Sustainable Habits and Routines to Minimize the Impact of Frequent Travel

By adopting sustainable lifestyle habits and routines, you can minimize the impact of frequent travel on your well-being and optimize your body's ability to adapt to changing time zones. These techniques will not only help you reduce the severity and duration of jet lag but also promote overall health and vitality.

1. Establish a Consistent Sleep Routine:

- Stick to a regular sleep schedule: Go to bed and wake up at the same time every day, even on weekends or non-travel days, to maintain a consistent sleep-wake pattern.

- Create a sleep-friendly environment: Ensure your bedroom is conducive to quality sleep by minimizing noise, controlling lighting, and maintaining a comfortable temperature.

- Wind down before bed: Establish a pre-sleep routine that includes relaxation techniques, such as reading, taking a warm bath, or practicing mindfulness, to signal to your body that it's time to sleep.

2. Optimize Your Nutrition:

- Eat a balanced diet: Consume a variety of nutrient-rich foods, including fruits, vegetables, whole grains, lean proteins, and healthy fats, to support your overall health and energy levels.

- Stay hydrated: Drink plenty of water throughout the day to maintain hydration, as dehydration can exacerbate jet lag symptoms.

- Limit caffeine and alcohol intake: Caffeine can disrupt sleep patterns, while alcohol can interfere with sleep quality. Use them in moderation or avoid them close to bedtime.

3. Incorporate Physical Activity:

- Engage in regular exercise: Regular physical activity not only promotes overall health but also helps regulate sleep patterns and increase daytime alertness.

- Exercise outdoors: Expose yourself to natural sunlight during the day, as it helps regulate circadian rhythms and enhances mood and energy levels.

- Stretch during travel: Perform gentle stretching exercises or practice yoga during long flights to promote blood circulation and reduce muscle stiffness.

4. Manage Stress and Relaxation:

- Practice stress management techniques: Incorporate stress-reducing activities into your daily routine, such as meditation, deep breathing exercises, or engaging in hobbies you enjoy.

- Schedule downtime: Prioritize relaxation and self-care by setting aside time for activities that help you unwind and rejuvenate, such as reading, listening to music, or taking a walk in nature.

5. Optimize Travel Strategies:

- Adjust sleep and meal times pre-travel: Gradually shift your sleep and meal times a few days before travel to align with your destination's time zone.

- Hydrate during travel: Drink plenty of water during flights to stay hydrated, as airplane cabins can be dehydrating.

- Utilize light exposure: Seek exposure to natural light upon arrival at your destination to help reset your internal body clock.

6. Consider Supplements and Natural Remedies:

- Melatonin: Consult with a healthcare professional about using melatonin supplements, which can help regulate sleep-wake cycles and mitigate the effects of jet lag.

- Herbal remedies: Explore natural remedies such as valerian root, chamomile, or lavender, which have calming properties that may support sleep and relaxation.

- Consult a healthcare professional: Before using any supplements or natural remedies, seek advice from a healthcare professional to ensure they are safe and appropriate for you.

Techniques for Integrating Travel and Time Zone Adjustments into a Healthy, Balanced Lifestyle

These are some techniques for managing travel-related disruptions and incorporating healthy habits that support your physical, mental, and emotional health. By implementing these strategies, you can navigate time zone adjustments and travel demands while staying true to your health and wellness goals.

1. Plan Ahead:

- Research your destination: Gain insight into the local culture, available food options, fitness facilities, and wellness activities at your destination. This will help you plan and make informed choices.

- Pack healthy essentials: Prepare travel-friendly snacks, water bottles, and any necessary supplements or medications to support your dietary and health needs during the journey.

- Create a travel itinerary: Organize your travel schedule, including flight times, layovers, and time zone changes. This will help you anticipate and plan for potential disruptions to your routine.

2. Prioritize Sleep and Rest:

- Stick to a sleep routine: Establish consistent sleep and wake-up times, even when traveling. This will help regulate your circadian rhythm and promote better sleep quality.

- Utilize sleep aids strategically: Consider using sleep aids such as earplugs, eye masks, or white noise machines to create a more comfortable sleep environment, especially during flights or in noisy hotel rooms.

- Allow for recovery time: When planning your itinerary, factor in rest days or buffer time to recuperate from long flights or adjust to time zone changes.

3. Maintain a Balanced Diet:

- Choose healthy food options: Opt for nutritious, whole foods whenever possible, including fruits, vegetables, lean proteins, and whole grains. Seek out local cuisine that aligns with your dietary preferences and goals.

- Practice portion control: Be mindful of portion sizes, especially when dining out or indulging in local specialties. Listen to your body's hunger and fullness cues to avoid overeating.

- Stay hydrated: Drink plenty of water throughout your journey to stay hydrated and support your overall well-being. Carry a reusable water bottle and refill it regularly.

4. Stay Active:

- Engage in physical activity: Incorporate movement into your travel routine by walking, stretching, or exploring your destination on foot. If possible, seek out local fitness facilities or outdoor activities that align with your interests.

- Exercise during layovers: Take advantage of airport facilities or nearby parks to engage in short workouts or stretching sessions during layovers. This can help combat stiffness and promote circulation.

- Embrace active sightseeing: Explore your destination through physical activities such as hiking, biking, or walking tours. This allows you to stay active while experiencing the local culture and attractions.

5. Manage Stress and Relaxation:

- Practice stress management techniques: Incorporate mindfulness exercises, deep breathing, or meditation into your daily routine to help manage stress and promote relaxation during travel.

- Create self-care rituals: Allocate time for activities that bring you joy and relaxation, such as reading, listening to music, taking baths, or practicing hobbies, even while on the go.

- Seek out relaxation amenities: Research hotels or accommodations that offer spa services, yoga classes, or wellness facilities. Taking advantage of these amenities can enhance your relaxation and rejuvenation during your trip.

6. Embrace Flexibility and Adaptability:

- Embrace the local culture: Immerse yourself in the local customs and traditions, including mealtimes and daily routines. This can help you adjust to the local time zone and embrace the destination fully.

- Be flexible with your schedule: Allow for spontaneity and adaptability in your travel plans. Sometimes the unexpected experiences can be the most rewarding, and being open to new opportunities can enhance your overall travel experience.

- Practice self-compassion: Remember that travel disruptions and time zone adjustments are inevitable. Be kind to yourself and practice self-care as you navigate these challenges. Focus on progress, not perfection.

Conclusion

Thriving in Any Time Zone - Your Path to Jet Lag Mastery

Congratulations! You have now journeyed through the pages of this book and gained valuable insights into understanding, managing, and overcoming the challenges of jet lag. Armed with expert strategies and practical techniques, you are well-equipped to thrive in any time zone and embrace a life of jet lag mastery.

Throughout this book, we explored the science behind jet lag and its effects on the body and mind. We delved into factors that contribute to the severity of jet lag symptoms, discussed pre-travel preparation strategies, and provided tips for optimizing your physical and mental state prior to travel. We then delved into in-flight strategies, ways to create a comfortable environment for better rest and recovery, and time zone transition techniques.

We examined the importance of adjusting sleep and meal times, improving sleep hygiene and incorporating relaxation techniques for better sleep quality. We also delved into the significance of nutrition and hydration in supporting energy and vitality during travel. Additionally, we explored recommendations for meals and snacks that aid in reducing jet lag symptoms and discussed active strategies for circadian rhythm adjustment.

We covered techniques for syncing your body's internal clock with the new time zone, and provided guidance on natural remedies, supplements, and productivity optimization strategies. We also discussed managing work or personal commitments during travel, long-term jet lag prevention and management, and techniques for integrating travel and time zone adjustments into a healthy, balanced lifestyle.

Now, armed with this comprehensive understanding and a toolbox of effective strategies, you have the power to conquer jet lag and unlock your potential to thrive in any time zone. By applying these insights and techniques, you can optimize your sleep, nourish your body, manage stress, and adapt to new time zones with ease.

Remember, jet lag mastery is not about eliminating travel challenges entirely. It is about embracing the journey and using the knowledge and tools at your disposal to navigate time zone changes and travel demands with grace and resilience. It is about taking care of yourself, prioritizing your well-being, and finding joy in the adventure of exploring new destinations.

Rise Above Jet Lag

As you embark on your future travels, remember the importance of preparation, flexibility, and self-care. Embrace the excitement of exploring new cultures and destinations, while also honoring your body's need for rest, nourishment, and rejuvenation. By finding harmony between your travel experiences and your well-being, you can truly thrive in any time zone.

Thank you for joining me on this transformative journey. I hope that this book has empowered you to take control of your travel experiences, conquer jet lag, and unlock your full potential in every aspect of your life. May you embark on future travels with renewed energy, vitality, and a deep sense of well-being. Here's to thriving in any time zone and embracing a life of jet lag mastery!

Safe travels and happy adventures!

www.ingramcontent.com/pod-product-compliance
Lightning Source LLC
Chambersburg PA
CBHW061352250726
48657CB00004B/1447